GROWING OLD

T. N. Rudd

*Didst thou see the thin hands of thy mother, held up as
  men sung
The low song of the nearly-departed, and heard her faint
  tongue
Joining in while it could to the witness, 'Let one more attest,
I have lived, seen God's hand thro' a lifetime, and all was
  for best . . .'*
Browning: Saul 9.15–18

SLG Press
Convent of the Incarnation
Fairacres Oxford

© THE SISTERS OF THE LOVE OF GOD 1988

Second Impression 1989

ISBN 0 7283 0120 2
ISSN 0307-1405

IN RECENT YEARS many books, pamphlets and articles have been published on the subject of retirement. These have explored adequately the physical, social and economic aspects of a situation which is being imposed on more and more people at a progressively earlier age. Many of these publications are excellent and of the greatest value to those about to retire as well as to those who have already done so. Unfortunately most of them confine themselves to the material aspects of retirement. They exclude the spiritual values which give life meaning, and consequently throw into undue prominence the rights of old people, and how to obtain them, with little or no emphasis on the responsibilities the retired person retains and how he can find fulfilment in life once work satisfactions have been withdrawn. They neglect the more difficult subject of work still to be done and contributions to the lives of others still to be made. The use of such publications is good, then, as far as they go— but they do not go far enough. They encourage one to be content with living on a plateau of life, all major achievement completed, with the remaining years devoted to enjoying the fruits of former harvests. The possibility of continued development is not considered, nor the frustration which is inherent in any situation where the only change envisaged is in a downward direction.

I believe that where these writings fail is in their lack of attention to the spiritual realm; they have little or nothing to say to the individual who is aware that 'man does not live by bread alone', or to the person who has unsatisfied religious needs. Since the religious instinct is deeply implanted in our human nature the need for a religious approach to life is more important than many writers will admit. Most of us are familiar with the words of C.G. Jung: ' Among all my patients in the second half of life—that is to say, over thirty-five—there has not been one whose problem in the last resort was not that of finding a religious outlook on life . . . and none of them has been really healed, who did not regain his religious outlook'. Indeed, he considers that many neuroses are caused by people blinding themselves to their own religious promptings 'because of a childish passion for rational enlightenment'. From a psychological perspective alone, then, it is not surprising that we grow old unsatisfactorily when our personalities are deprived of such a basic need. To go through the later stages of life without any thought of the meaning of life and author of our existence is a situation fraught with danger.

This consideration explains the title of this pamphlet, *Growing Old with God*. The phrase is suggested by its opposite, 'growing old *without* God', which seems to be the position of many elderly people who end their lives in sadness and despondency. The suicide rate in the older age groups is a subject of great concern to psychiatrists; it is, however, only the tip of the iceberg which conceals a major problem of old age, the fear and unhappiness in those who have made valued contributions to life and who deserve the opportunity to live happily and continue in the service of others. Many of us well advanced in age may feel 'it is toward evening and the day is now far spent', but this does not apply to those entering retirement. With social policies advocating universal, compulsory retirement at ever earlier ages, men and women are facing retired lives with unimpaired vitality and the prospect of perhaps thirty years (up to one-third of the total life span) stretching before them. It is a new situation, both for the individual and for society and one which requires recognizing our assumptions and perhaps adopting new attitudes. Even if one does not consider oneself as old, the prospect of old age is there on the horizon and one is bound to regard oneself as having left a high point of life. But when the prospect of old age is daunting it is good to remind oneself of Jung's dictum that 'a human being would certainly not grow to seventy or eighty years old if this longevity had no meaning for the species to which he belongs'.

A willingness to grow further

I think it is necessary for each one of us to recognize retirement is a watershed in our lives; it divides our earlier physically productive years where our energies were spent on making our way in the world from our later years when we consolidate what we have so far achieved. To pass successfully through progressive stages of life—each of which has its advantages and disadvantages and its unique contribution to make to the maturation of personality—demands a reorientation; it demands a willingness to grow further and to leave behind accustomed patterns of thought and adopt new attitudes and responsibilities. Life can no longer be lived, at least successfully, with attitudes which were healthy and necessary when we were young. In this readjustment many people need help, which is not always readily available, even from doctors and the clergy, who after all, face similar problems in their own lives.

At the outset, we must get our thoughts straight about retirement, irrespective of the age at which it is imposed on us. The first necessity is to avoid resentment and the feeling of being hurt because we have been unfairly superseded by a younger person. Cognate with this resentment is that of self-depreciation, the feeling that one has been thrown on the scrap-heap and forced into an old age that is both useless and depressing. Why do we feel worthless? Is this not an example of the damage that can be done by the competitive attitudes which tended to dominate our working years? Such attitudes have been double-edged weapons which, while perhaps advancing us in life, did so at the cost of damaged personalities and diminished happiness. Unless we can recognize and re-evaluate the mistaken assumption that we are now worth less as people than we were when we began preparing for a career we will not be ready to adjust to this new stage of life. We may miss the opportunity of discovering our years in retirement as a time when losses can be made good and peace of mind attained, perhaps for the first time.

Frustration and restlessness

The foundation as well as the fruit of our reassessment of ourselves as retired persons, as I suggested earlier, is in the spiritual realm, and it is significant that during these years many begin to recognize the importance of the religious and philosophical insights which seemed irrelevant in earlier life. Some discover a need for religion naturally, some after prolonged suffering, others perhaps after a Jungian psychoanalysis. They begin to understand that man is a religious animal, and as such feels frustrated and unhappy when his religious needs are not satisfied. It is not surprising that we grow old unsatisfactorily when our personalities are deprived of such an important component. Would we expect a car to function well with only half its cylinders working? Perhaps it can only be during the years when we are no longer distracted by the demands of a young family and a career that we will be forced to recognize and integrate various aspects of our personalities, various rejected attitudes, including our religious needs, which thus far have not claimed our attention. But the happiness and constructive use of the years of our retirement may depend on our response to the inner promptings of our hearts.

Thou hast made us

We have now entered that part of life where our achievements and conflicts will be largely within ourselves, something the ancient and classical writers called the *psychomachia*, the battle of the mind. Now through a deepening awareness of our need for God, and the expression of our relationship with him in our relationships with others and in every detail of our life, we will realize that this need is also part of God's need for us and his desire for our growth and healing. Increasingly as we recognize the work of God in our lives, we will also know his love and gain confidence for the interior and exterior work awaiting us. Above all, as we see a purpose in our struggle, in the restlessness and lack of satisfaction in our lives, we will see that even our present needs are within God's loving purpose. Recovering our sense of direction, though difficult, should not prove impossible. God, who himself is wholeness, has designed wholeness for all creation. We are, most of us, born with the potential for a full life—which, however, few of us manage to achieve. But recognizing, accepting and acting upon the knowledge of parts of our personality which for one reason or another we have repressed (what a Jungian psychologist would call the 'shadow side' of our personalities gone underground) constitutes a considerable and valuable part of our growth.

This work of growth is one that is asked of us at all stages of our life, and the problems of arrested development are not confined to childhood or adolescence. People who fail to grow in accord with nature's demands, who 'get stuck' as it were, are usually neither happy nor easy to live with. We find people fixated at 'sixth form level', elderly women clinging to the role of mother of a growing family, and even captains of industry who in retirement adhere to outdated attitudes which earlier brought success. Men sometimes reject attitudes of charitable love or sympathy which they regard as womanish, and thus develop into over-masterful personalities, concerned only with success, power and domination. Women, in their turn, may avoid or fear a managerial role, choosing to remain as pampered sex objects. Neither of these approaches stands the test of time and the personalities concerned tend to 'run out of steam' in the fifth or sixth decade. They form the mass of discontented elderly women and bored grumbling old men. Younger people in whom the retardation may be less obvious are dissatisfied with the pointlessness of their lives and plague their families with unsocial behaviour and perpetually seek, from Eastern mysticism or elsewhere, some magic formula which will set them free from their frustrations. It may be that the years of retirement are the time when along with our recognition of our need for God we will see that facing our needs and frustrations is a means of gaining true freedom and is part of God's plan for us. The words of St Augustine at the beginning of his *Confessions* which recount the work of God in his own life, 'Thou has made us for thyself and our hearts are restless till they rest in Thee', will become words we can make our own, words speaking of God at work in our lives and of his love.

The medicament of immortality

During our retirement years we are building on strengths and weaknesses that existed previously. I can therefore speak only in general terms about problems of adjustment because there is such a wide variety of factors to be considered. We are concerned with both men and women and with social, economic and emotional factors. The attitude to retirement and the degree of its acceptance is paramount and this is determined in large part by achievements and satisfactions gained during working years—though our acceptance of retirement does mean putting aside these satisfactions. The problems of marital adjustment, when they exist, cannot be avoided as easily as before. Partnerships which were manageable when the couple were absent from each other during the working day, may go into strain when the situation is changed. One remembers the remark of the wife of the newly-retired man, who said she had married him 'for love but not for lunch'!

One can also think of the boredom and loneliness of those who have developed few interests and have not learned to make and keep friends. Some people are more prepared to enjoy their retirement than others. The perpetual student, the gardener and the DIY enthusiast will continue to find satisfaction most of the year, given necessary health, while the devoted housewife and mother or grandmother may be kept quite busy, even when she has given up a professional or business life. But in spite of this, many people do face an empty existence and for them the long leisure of retirement is difficult. Clearly there is no one single answer, and as well as using our leisure during retirement constructively, there is value in looking ahead and preparing for these years. Each one of us must seek an answer for himself, and preferably before retirement overtakes him, and in this lies the great value of pre-retirement courses and counselling.

We must realize though, that even if we are relatively well prepared, there is no way to shield ourselves from having to accept the real difficulties encountered during these years. I believe they can be happy years, years of growth, but they are also years of suffering. The later stages of life are generally overclouded by the multiple losses to which old age is liable. These cover every aspect of our lives, including loss of home through separation and bereavement. Apt to affect us at all times of life, these blows fall most heavily in old age. But is there no hope? I believe there is. This is why I emphasize the importance of the spiritual realm; these are problems for which a wholly 'this-world' approach has no answer. If our present existence is all we have, the uncertainties and fears of later life may well be devastating. Their only cure may lie in the medicament of immortality, the *athanasias pharmakon* of the ancient spiritual writers. The remedy is in the hope of God's loving purpose for us throughout and beyond our earthly life.

Images of old age

Common stereotypes of old age are based on the physical and economic decline of these years. Sophocles, writing in the fifth century BC laments,

> And sealing the sum of trouble, doth tottering Age draw nigh,
> Whom friends and kinsfolk fly,
> Age, upon whom redouble all sorrows under the sky.

Today's popular image is less starkly tragic but hardly more inviting. The years of retirement are viewed as a pleasantly useless time when we qualify for receiving patronage and handouts—free travel passes and reduced entrance charges ('children and O.A.Ps.'). Old age is seen as a time for receiving gifts, with no emphasis on gifts also being given, no emphasis on a continuing contribution to community and family life, on the essential role the old play in society. This 'bingo' image does nothing but downgrade the idea of old people in the eyes of others, and what is worse, in their own eyes.

The concept of the elders of the tribe maintaining the cultural and moral values has become entirely alien to us, or so it would seem. But do we not depend on the achievements of generations who have gone before us, and do we not respect those whose sometimes heroic example we would like to follow? Scripture alone presents us with many figures that can serve as an illustration. The First Reading at a Mass on the Feast of Saints Thomas More and John Fisher is the story of old Eleazer, the grand old man of the Maccabees, who during the persecution of the Jews in the second century BC gave up his life rather than set a bad example.

> Eleazar, one of the foremost teachers of the Law, a man already advanced in years and of most noble appearance, was being forced to open his mouth wide to swallow pig's flesh. Those in charge of the impious banquet, . . . took him aside and privately urged him to have meat brought of a kind he could properly use, prepared by himself, and only pretend to eat the portions of sacrificial meat prescribed by the king. 'Such pretence,' he said, 'does not square with our time of life; many young people would suppose that Eleazar at the age of ninety had conformed to the foreigners' way of life, and because I had played this part for the sake of a paltry brief spell of life might themselves be led

astray on my account; I should only bring defilement and disgrace on my old age. . . .Therefore if I am man enough to quit this life here and now I shall prove myself worthy of my old age, and I shall have left the young a noble example of how to make a good death, eagerly and generously, for the venerable and holy laws.' With these words he went straight to the block. (2 Maccabees 6.18–28 JB)

The heroic stand of Eleazer is only a dramatic instance of the responsibilities of the elderly. It is the Church's teaching that all God's people live in fulfilment of his plan for the world, and that God maintains us in life so that his eternal purpose can be effected. This not only explains the sacrifice of Eleazer, and of other martyrs through the ages like Thomas More and John Fisher, but affirms the value of every human life.

The situation of the elderly is thus, by no means, a purely receptive one; there are contributions to be made, not only to society, without which our world would be poorer, but also in the development of the individual personality, what Teilhard de Chardin and C.G. Jung have each called 'making the soul'. Spiritual contributions do affect the health, or lack of it, of a society (even when we cannot explain how this works), and even when the contributions we make are strictly social and material, they nevertheless possess a spiritual significance for the giver. The Christian approaches life with one hand stretched out to God and the other to his fellow man.

Many of our great charitable organizations are so dependent on the contributions of retired people that, if their voluntary labour was withdrawn, survival would be difficult. Cathedrals and parish churches of all denominations depend heavily on volunteers for cleaning the building and acting as guides; such services, generously given, are valuable not only for the churches but for the individuals concerned. An even more important contribution an older person can make is to family life, what may be properly called 'the role of the grandparent in modern society'. We have already considered the example of Eleazar, the archetypal grandfather, the embodiment and guardian of the religious and moral values of his people. Generally the role of today's grandparent is much more mundane—though what would young parents do without the aid of grandparents for baby-sitting?—but many young families need the support of their own parents in all kinds of ways, and it is also important for children to have this contact with members of an older generation.

Hidden works of service

As life advances and physical strength fails, even the kinds of unpaid work we have been able to do will become more limited, even regular church attendance on Sunday may become difficult. Apart then from the private life of prayer, and for some, visits from a priest bringing Holy Communion, our Christian witness will consist in our immediate relationships and household tasks performed in a spirit of love. In such humble and hidden works of service, motivation is the important thing. All our actions are performed in the sight of God and for God. Jung speaks of the way in which we do the peeling of potatoes and washing of dirty plates as our 'service to the object'. The value of such work in our spiritual life has been described in the writings of the greatest teachers of the life of prayer, including Teresa of Avila who said she found God walking among the pots and pans of her kitchen, and another Carmelite, Brother Lawrence (the author of *The Practice of the Presence of God*) who said that he found himself as near to God in the lowly cleaning tasks in the monastic scullery, as at the moment of the elevation of the Host at Mass. George Herbert also speaks of the same awareness of God's presence in his hymn,

> Teach me, my God and King,
> In all things thee to see;
> And what I do in anything
> To do it as for thee!

Whatever we do in the presence of God can become a joyous service to God and a contribution towards the perfection of his work.

Prayer it seems, is very much a part of the specific work of the Christian in old age. Even in youth and middle age when physical activity is unimpaired we should develop our two-fold vocation to a life of prayer and love, but this is a special privilege of the older person, as well as his required contribution. Our long life should have taught us a sensitivity to spiritual influences—that some people lack this awareness and deny that such influences exist does not mean that our own feelings on this subject are delusions. As we look over our life, we are bound to be aware of difficult situations which were resolved happily, surely through the prayers of our friends and fellow Christians. While being grateful for these, we should also learn that we should, in our turn, pray for others in their need.

Not all of us can be like Anna, the daughter of Phanuel, who with Simeon greeted the Holy Child and his Mother at the Presentation in the Temple (cf. Luke 2.22–38). This eighty-four-year old widow 'did not depart from the temple, worshipping with fasting and prayer night and day.' But her consecrated life and the fulfilment of the promise made to Simeon 'that he should not see death before he had seen the Lord's Christ' are far better images of the life and witness of an elderly Christian than what we think when we are tempted to say, whether we mean it or not, 'I'm just a poor old body, not worth bothering about'.

The exercise of love

Prayer, then, is one of the responsibilities of these years, and also the work of loving—loving which is not just a matter of feelings, but of doing. When the time of physical activity is past and we are confined to the house, to one floor, or even to our bedroom, the functions of praying and loving become even more important, even more revealing. At the moment when death seems imminent, we are more likely to remember not our very minor successes in life, but how much we have loved. As John of the Cross says in the *Spiritual Canticle*, 'Now I guard no flock nor have I now other office, For now my exercise is in loving alone.' He comments that the speaker in the stanza says

> all the things wherewith my soul and my body are provided: memory, understanding and will, inward and outward senses, desires of the sensual part and of the spiritual part. All these work in love and for the sake of love, so that all that I do I do with love and all that I suffer I suffer with the pleasure of love. (Stanza XXVIII, trans. Peers)

This exercise of love is that means by which we can help to neutralize, to absorb, some of the conflict and hatred in today's world. We can still try to show readiness to be pleased with life and patient under whatever befalls, seeing the finger of God in everything. Joyfulness, even in great disability, is the sign of a mature spirit, growing into God, and a measure of the love we have given out may be glimpsed at times in the pleasure our family and friends take in visiting us.

There are, of course, hazards and temptations during retirement years which take away our joy, but what age is free of them? Some are not new to us, but are especially troublesome because of our altered circumstances. Perhaps the most formidable impediment to joy is what was anciently called *accidie*, the sin of sloth. It is now called 'boredom', but what it entails is a sense of the futility of existence and of further effort. This is not only a miserable state, but it is quite wrong because it is contrary to the Church's teaching that our continuance in life is the will of God. As I said earlier, old age is no time for 'getting stuck' and resisting further development; it is rather the beginning of a metamorphosis, the end of which we are unable to see this side of the grave. Feeling that we are finished in life generates an unnecessary querulousness and petulance and we must resist this. It is quite unrelated to our situation in life, and it may make our friends avoid, rather than seek, our company.

Fears and anxiety

Something more should be said, however, about the fears and anxieties of later life. These come in many different forms, some of which lie within the purely medical or psychiatric fields. Some fears are clearly associated with all the hazards, social, economic, physical and spiritual, which old age has to face, and these are quite realistic fears. Some needless fears, however, reflect a lack of faith which a firmer trust in God would have allayed. Remember how our Lord said to Peter, 'O man of little faith, why did you doubt?' (Mat. 14.31). Apart from such fears, however, there is the terrible free-floating anxiety which affects many older people, and for which many resort to tranquillizing drugs. This is a general sense of fearfulness, sometimes described as 'butterflies in the stomach', and it is responsible for the unnecessary prescribing of sedative tablets and sleeping pills; 'unnecessary', I say, since the cause may be spiritual, not physical. Whereas the major fears of life, often associated with true mental depression are a form of psychiatric illness, free-floating anxiety is quite different. Theologically speaking, such a lack of faith would be considered a sin. It is important to realize this, because tranquillisers can never cure lack of faith though they may temporarily mask the symptoms. Also they do not overcome the paralysis of action which such fears produce, nor do they strengthen and encourage those whose lives are becoming more and more narrow. What may be needed is some form of Christian ministry, perhaps confession, absolution and ghostly counsel to put us right. Only by asking and receiving from God an increased trust in his mercy and providence can souls reach, even in old age, their full potential. We must take to ourselves the full meaning of our Lord's comforting words, 'Fear not, little flock, for it is your Father's good pleasure to give you the kingdom.' (Luke 12.32) It is only with a full trust in God that we can 'put away childish things' and experience the joy of retirement and old age which should be our inheritance as sons of our Father who is in Heaven.

Preserving our faith depends in part at least, in developing an adult image of God, an image in keeping with our own level of maturity. Children may think of God as a long-bearded ancestor sitting upon a throne, and Christ as the loving shepherd, carrying lamb and crook. But as life progresses we realize that these images are expressing a mystery beyond images, expressing a truth about Christ whom we begin to understand as absolute love seeking love in return, and God himself as intangible, absolute, and in some ways unknowable. Growing beyond our childish concepts may make our adult faith more difficult, perhaps a little distant unless sustained by experience, especially a sense of God's indwelling presence, but it is a means of receiving not our own image of God, but God himself. We are called to a life of faith, and as our faith is strengthened our childish fears will be taken up into a larger sense that God, who has brought us safe thus far, will not abandon us. An expression of a mature faith can be found in the words of Job,

> I know that my redeemer liveth, and that he shall stand at the latter day upon the earth: and though after my skin worms destroy this body, yet in my flesh shall I see God. (Job 19.25 AV)

Spiritual reading

Much has been written about faulty nutrition as a factor in unsatisfactory ageing, but undernourishment can occur in mental and spiritual spheres as well as in the physical. When we say the Lord's Prayer, we ask to be given our daily bread, not always considering what this consists of, or from whence it comes. The phrase following our request for bread is 'and forgive us our trespasses'. This suggests to me that part of our sustenance is meant to be on the spiritual level, and that the prayer makes this provision because of our liability to neglect our spiritual food or to undervalue it. I have already described some of the ways in which our vital spiritual nourishment comes to us: through seeking to respond to the will of God in everything that we do; through the sacraments, especially the Holy Eucharist; and in prayer in all its forms. Those requiring specific guidance about these areas of their life should consult a priest, pastor or spiritual director.

Another important kind of spiritual nourishment is that of spiritual reading, which we may have overlooked when we were younger, or at least until recent years when so many varied and inexpensive books on spirituality are available. It seems to me that regular study of the Bible and familiarity with the Book of Common Prayer or the Missal has fallen off since post-Reformation days. If this is so, we are much impoverished thereby since all Christian study and the life of prayer require a thorough grounding in Scripture; and a proper understanding of other spiritual writings assumes this knowledge. The Bible, then, should be a regular part of our spiritual diet. We might also find ourselves greatly enriched by becoming acquainted or re-acquainted with religious classics like the *Confessions* of St Augustine or *The Practice of the Presence of God*, which I have mentioned previously, or perhaps the fourteenth century mystics, especially Julian of Norwich, or the sixteenth century Carmelites, Teresa of Avila and John of the Cross—though they are difficult for untrained minds. Most spiritual classics are classics because many generations have found them rewarding, and often they are more approachable than you might expect. Modern religious book shops are now offering a wide variety of books on spirituality, some of them selections from the classics arranged as daily readings which will serve as an introduction to an author as well as being very good for devotional use. (A good example of such is the 'Enfolded in Love' series published by Darton Longman and Todd.)

Our spiritual diet can be quite varied, and will include as well as the classics, one or more modern writers on spirituality such as Thomas Merton, Gerald Vann, William Johnston, or Robert Llewelyn, the last a specialist on Julian of Norwich. To this very varied list, we might well add Rabbi Lionel Blue, whose deep but down-to-earth approach to religion can illumine dark corners of our spiritual house, as it were. All of these writers and many others have something to say to us that we would do well to heed. Perhaps we should also seek advice as to our reading, lest our first choice is so unfortunate that we conclude that spiritual reading is not for us. Perhaps I can offer this word of caution on reading the lives of the saints: valuable and interesting as some of these can be, it is possible to treat such material with a detached attitude appropriate to a work of literature or history. We should not read the lives of the saints in the same detached manner, however, because these books are describing Christians like ourselves, and we seek to add them to our diet of spiritual reading as an example of Christian life to enlarge and challenge our own witness.

Today we hear a lot about 'convenience foods', which are sometimes lacking in nutritional value. Convenience foods for the mind present an even greater danger. The media, particularly newspapers and television, present particular hazards and are foremost as time-wasters in old age. This is a particular temptation now when one is bored and tired. Even crossword puzzles of the more difficult kinds, although good mental stimulants, can waste our days if we become devoted to them and give them a lot of time when we could be better employed. Selective television watching can be good, but it too can become a bad habit, a crutch. This can also be true of having the radio on all day long—without even listening to it! However, finding ways of using our long leisure, when one is almost confined to a chair presents a real difficulty, I know. Writing letters of cheer and comfort to our friends is a splendid activity, when we are able to write, or perhaps we can make an occasional phone call. Giving thanks for the beauty and goodness that surround us, or offering prayer for our suffering or the suffering of others who lack such blessings, can become a regular part of our life. Even simple thinking about the goodness of God and how best to respond to him in our daily actions is an excellent habit and can amount to prayer. There is, indeed, only a small step between this kind of thinking and simple 'meditation'. If our minds have, in earlier life, been familiar with psalms and hymns embodying sound Christian teaching, we will be supplied with excellent material to set our thoughts on things of God even when we have no books at hand, but fortunately we can also always add treasures to this spiritual storehouse.

Unknown country

At this point perhaps it will be useful to consider where we now stand in viewing our life in retirement, and especially the direction we appear to be taking in our journey through the last years of our life. Learning to adjust to retirement and old age takes time and patience, but as we succeed, we become happier and able to accept with humility a new and challenging adventure which can bring much joy. New satisfactions are available to us in the contributions still possible in our circumstances. We should have found out, too, that service to our fellows, if it is to be truly effective needs to be based on our duty to God.

I trust we are also learning to adjust to our diminishments, and to accept them, as far as is possible, as part of God's plan for us—not only those already affecting us, but also those which may assail us in the future. For this difficult task we need all the faith we can muster, hope which can pierce the curtain of death to whatever lies beyond, and love; love for those around us, for the whole of groaning and suffering creation, and for God himself who alone understands why things are as they are. For this, much prayer is needed, but through prayer even these adjustments will bear fruit and can generate joy in ourselves and those around us—even in the most unlikely conditions.

We are beginning to travel into unknown country and the terrain will include rocky and steep paths, and perhaps a desert.

This country is likely to include bereavements, and for many the loss of a marriage partner will mean a change in living-pattern. Help can be gained through bereavement counselling, which has now attained a sound level. It is also comforting to remember that earthly love and all we receive in life are gifts from God and are shadows of what we will receive in the life to come.

Loss of home, physical disability and admission as a long-stay resident into a hospital or residential home are other major adjustments to be faced. Residents in such institutions are not always the recipients of an ideal level of care, they often have much to put up with from the humiliations and restrictions that come their way, which is why our learning to accept these experiences is so important. Although the quality of care has improved immeasurably in the last decades, much still remains to be done. Even now, not every trained nurse fully understands the needs of elderly patients; how then can we expect more from untrained nursing assistants, much of whose loving and devoted attention derives from their own natural sympathy and Christian charity. We do well to pray for our doctors and nurses. Perhaps we should remember that it is the patients who need our prayers even more.

Yet as Christians we are bound to remember that suffering has at any age a spiritual value which may be an essential part of God's plan for perfecting the soul. Neither the patients nor those concerned about them have cause to deny that this part of the journey into an unknown country is part of God's plan for us. Therefore attempting to curtail God's plan for us, by any form of artificial termination of life, is completely excluded. Pain and suffering can and should be relieved. Many demands for euthanasia arise because such help has not been effectively given. Most Health Districts now have medical consultants, expert in pain relief and terminal care, and their advice should be sought, where necessary, through the family doctor.

Death

Shadowing us all the time in our last years is the thought of death, and indeed, death itself. St Paul refers to death as the last enemy to be overcome (I Cor. 15.26)—though later in that same wonderful chapter he says that 'Death is swallowed up in victory'. This is theological language. On the human plane, the experience of death, especially in old age, is less an enemy than a friend. St Francis speaks of 'Sister Death, who brings peace and rest to the weary soul'. Certainly for the Christian (and also for other 'People of the Book'—devout Jews and Moslems) the event of death should bring no fear; while, as I said before, the pain of dying and any preceding suffering can be alleviated by proper physical and spiritual care.

So far as we can judge, the act of dying seldom creates alarm or pain, and those of us who have approached the frontiers of life and have returned safely may have been altered by the experience, but have not been terrified. Weakness and weariness may even make us prefer death to life, as St Paul and St Catherine of Siena both confess. This is a matter best left to the Lord. We must await our time in patience, seeking meanwhile to complete our life task.

The following stanzas from a poem by St Peter Damian* explain the purpose of the struggle of our last years. The image of the exile returning to his own country describes our own journey:

> For the fount of life undying
>   Once the parched mind did thirst,
> Cramped within its carnal prison,
>   Sought the soul its bonds to burst.
> Struggling, gliding, soaring free,
> Comes back the exile to its own country.
>
> Cleansed from all its dregs, the body
>   With the spirit knows no war
> For the mind and flesh made spirit
>   One in thought and feeling are
> Deep their peace and their enjoying
> From all shame and scandal far.

We should be grateful that the years of retirement and old age are given to us to enable us to carry out this process of mind

---

* Helen Waddell: *THE WANDERING SCHOLARS*, London: Constable and Co. Ltd., 1927, p. 86.

and flesh becoming spirit. All opportunities for service, all suffering and diminishment serve to prepare us for endless life. The leisure of retirement is given to us to enable us to grow into full maturity and to complete our earthly task. We should therefore accept this opportunity and use it fully with joy and thankfulness, knowing that the work of the last years allotted to us is part of God's plan for our lives. Every day, indeed, every experience, is important. Dr Michael O'Donnell, the medical writer and broadcaster, relates that a patient once wrote to him,

> It's odd how illness made my life worth living. How awful it would have been if, instead of getting ill, I'd been hit by a bus and extinguished immediately, without ever learning what life really had to offer.

Let us remember always that the last years of our life are worth living. Even when our journey leads us into the desert, when through weakness or infirmity we can contribute little to our fellows, or even care for ourselves, we are always in God's love and love remains our last gift to God and to others. Those of us who have been privileged to witness the holy death of someone who has lost the faculties of sight, hearing and movement can testify to the mystery of love and the mystery of death. We have understood in a new way the words of the Prophet Isaiah: 'The wilderness and the solitary place shall be glad for them; and the desert shall rejoice, and blossom as the rose' (Isa. 35.1).